7 Food Habits

for

Weight Loss Forever

by Subodh Gupta

First Edition January 2008

Copyright @2008 by Subodh Gupta

ISBN 978-0-9556882-0-1

Published by
Subodh Gupta
+44(0)7966275913
Head office: London (UK)
Email: info@subodhgupta.com
Website: www.subodhgupta.com

Publisher Note:
The reader should not regard the recommendation in this book as substitute advice of a qualified medical practitioner. The aim of this book is to create awareness among the masses about unhealthy food habits. The information does not endorse any particular brand.

Acknowledgements

I am grateful to my parents and all my teachers who taught me at various stages of my life & shared with me their wisdom.

Content

Introduction:

According to department of health (UK), "*In 2005, 22% of English men and 24% of women were classified as obese*"[1] and if we continue as per past trend, Obesity will be increasing at alarming rate effecting nation health seriously. "*Over the last 25 years, the number of people classed as either overweight or obese in England has tripled*" according to UK government Foresight program.[2]

Obesity is increasing not only in England but in the whole developed world. You would be surprised to know that "*Scotland is the second fattest nation in the developed world, behind America*" and "*Percentage of obese members of the population around the world, United States: 32.2, Scotland: 25.5, Mexico: 24.2, England: 22.5, Canada: 22.4, Greece: 21.9*".[3]

USA, UK, Canada are certainly among the economically wealthy countries where medical science is very advance and these countries spend millions of dollars on research. Literacy level of people is also very high as compared to most of the other nations on this planet. That means people are educated and understand what is right and healthy for them.

But then the point is: why the obesity level is so high considering the fact that *obesity is one of the major reasons for various diseases like heart disease, diabetes, back pain, cancer, arthritis and breathlessness, etc?*

Are our day to day eating habits good enough?

Most of the overweight people whom I interact tell me that they eat sensibly. Now the question is: if most of the people eat sensibly then why they are overweight and why there are so many deaths which are linked with our day to day eating habits?

According to American Cancer society *"Cancer accounts for nearly one-quarter of deaths in the United States, exceeded only by heart diseases"*.[4]In 2004, there were 553,888 cancer deaths in the US (23.1% of all death).

Heart disease accounts for 653486 deaths which is about 27.2% of all death in USA. *That means heart and cancer related death accounted more than 50 % of all death in USA in 2004.*

Similarly let's have a look at some of the statistics in UK.

According to Cancer research UK, *"One in four (26%) of all deaths in the UK are caused by cancer. There were 153,491 cancer deaths in the UK in 2005"*.[5]

You might be wondering why I am quoting so many statistics about cancer/ heart disease along with obesity.

The point is most of human body diseases like cancer and heart disease are linked with our food which we eat. *If people are eating healthy food then how can there be more than 50 % death from heart and cancer diseases?*

If we correct our eating habits then not only we would have perfect body weight but we would certainly get rid of most of diseases which are killing most of the western nations.

Managing perfect body weight is not a complicated rocket science. Our body is made up of food which we eat during our day to day life. If we are overweight or obese at the moment then one thing is certain that the food which we eat is not good.

This book has 2 parts.

First Part of this book contains knowledge and explores various food habits which have become part of our daily life. Understanding of these food habits can help you to prepare your mind to take action for achieving perfect body weight and health.

The Second Part contains tables to record your daily food habits and to note down your improvement. I strongly recommend everybody to follow the seven food habits as described in this book for 6 weeks and you will be amazed to see that how easily you could lose the extra body fat.

In the end I would like to say that healthy food habits will certainly lead you to good health and perfect body weight forever.

May all being be healthy.
Subodh Gupta

"He who does not know food, how can he understand the diseases of man?"

- Hippocrates, the father of medicine (460-357 B.C.)

Part 1
7 Food Habits

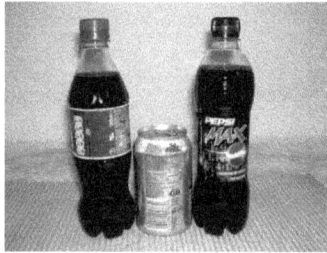

Some of the cola brand products can have **210 calories** in each 500 ml bottle along with **53 g of sugar**, flavouring (including caffeine) and phosphoric acid, while other brand products may have less calories and sugar but high amount of **Sweeteners,** Colour, **Preservative** (sodium Benzoate), **Citric acid** along with **Phosphoric acid**.

Food Habit No 1

Carbonated drinks

If I tell you there is something which most of us drink, everyday, round the globe and it may results in:

- Gaining weight

- Loss of tooth enamel

- More possibility of bone fracture for little girls

- Increased risk of osteoporosis

- Damaging your DNA cell and

Last but not the least it contains pesticides and traces of cancer causing elements as well.

Would you like to drink it?

Of course not but we drink it and guess how much?
....

As per figure published in Center for Science in the public interest (CSPI) website about consumption of carbonated soft drink in America *"companies annually produce enough soda pop to provide 557, 12-ounce cans, 52.4 gallons-to every man, woman and child"*.[6] (198.33 litre per person per year, that is almost equal to *more than half litre per day per person*, 1US gallon = 3.785 litre).

Drinking habit of soft drinks in UK is also not better. *"More than 5,560 million litres of carbonated soft drinks are consumed every year in the UK."*[7]

Let's consider at present UK population is approximately about 60 millions. That means each person in UK drinks about 92.66 litres per year.

It is definitely surprising. It seems that people in America and UK drink carbonated soft drinks in place of milk and water.

Welcome to the world of carbonated drinks.

Let's have a look on various researches which have been done over the years about the impact of carbonated drinks on human health.

Sugar Sweetened Drink and Child Obesity

You will be surprised to know that carbonated soft drinks are the largest single source of calories in American people diet, about seven percent of daily calories intake.

These soft drinks are not calorie-free. An average can of soda has carbonic or phosphoric acid and some have up to 50 mg of caffeine along with about 140 calories.

Many soft drinks (including fizzy and sweetened soft drinks) contain a lot of sugar, approximately 40-50 grams. These drinks are said to have lots of 'empty calories' – they can result in putting on extra weight and don't have much nutritional value.

"A child's odds of becoming obese increase by 60 percent with each additional daily serving of sugar-sweetened drinks". [8] (This was the conclusion of a recent study from the Department of Medicine at Children's Hospital in Boston and the Harvard School of Public Health).

Cola and Human teeth

Nobody wants to lose their teeth and people spent hundreds of pounds each in country like UK for teeth related issues.

What do you think can damage your teeth?

You might be shocked by the answer once you read the following information.

"Tooth decay happens when teeth are attacked by acid, and this can happen in two ways. Acid attacks can happen as a result of plaque bacteria acting on the sugars in our diet, or as a direct result of the acids in food dissolving away the enamel on the

16

surfaces of our teeth. As carbonated soft drinks tend to contain high amounts of both sugars and acids, they're the worst possible combination for dental health."[7]

Sipping the soft drink prolongs contact between our teeth and the "acid bath" which we give them without being aware.

Along with soft drinks, sports drinks and energy drinks are also responsible for tooth decay.

Wondering how…?

Because, most colas contain one or more acids, usually phosphoric and citric acids and sports beverages also contain organic acids which are also known to break down calcium.

The carbonic or phosphoric acid dissolves the calcium out of the enamel and it results into wide scale destruction.

Do you know that Cola beverage have the capacity to dissolve the human teeth?

Surprised, ok then read on the following.

According to an article by Mike Adams on News target titled: "The health effects of drinking soda - quotes from the experts" William Duffy
The doctor speaking in these dialogs is, Dr. McCay, the nutritionist at the Naval Medical Research Institute.

"I was amazed to learn," he testified, "that the beverage contained substantial amounts of phosphoric acid. . . . At the Naval Medical Research Institute, we put human teeth in a cola beverage and found they softened and started to dissolve within a short period… The acidity of cola beverages ... is about the same as vinegar. The sugar content masks the acidity, and children little realize they are drinking this strange mixture of phosphoric acid, sugar, caffeine, colouring, and flavouring matter."[9]

What are you thinking now??? Anyway, I have lots more for you to read and the following information is to the point.

Soft Drinks and Risk Of Osteoporosis

As per liquid candy *"Frequent consumption of soft drinks may also increase the risk of osteoporosis — especially in people who drink soft drinks instead of calcium-rich milk. Dental experts continue to urge that people drink less soda pop, especially between meals, to prevent tooth decay (due to the sugars) and dental erosion (due to the acids)"*.[6]

Cola and bone fracture:

Do you know that cola drinks have been linked to bone fracture?

According to an article published by Grace Wyshak, associate professor in the Departments of Biostatistics and Population and International Health at Harvard School of Public Health published in June 2000 issue *"Active girls who drink cola drinks are five times more likely to have had bone fractures than girls who don't drink soda pop"*.[10]

Another research…

Would you consider taking risk of damaging your DNA cell???

According to an article by Martin Hickman *titled* "caution : Some soft drinks may seriously harm your health: Experts link additive to cell damage " published on the Independent news website : "*A new health scare erupted over soft drinks last night amid evidence they may cause serious cell damage. Research from a British university suggests a common preservative found in drinks such as Fanta and Pepsi Max has the ability to switch off vital parts of DNA.*"[11]

Another research…

Cancer chemical found in British soft drinks

According to news published on BBC News 24 in Health section "*Traces of a cancer-causing chemical have been found in British soft drinks at eight times the level permitted in drinking water, BBC News has learned*".[12]

Another Study…

Pesticide in Soft drinks

According to Centre for Science and Environment (CSE)
"*The 2006 CSE study tests 57 samples of 11 soft drink brands, from 25 different manufacturing plants of Coca-Cola and PepsiCo, spread over 12 states. The study finds pesticide residues in all samples; it finds a cocktail of 3-5 different pesticides in all samples*".[13]

Now the interesting part of the story is that rather than improving the quality of soft drinks in India, Soft drinks companies hired "intelligent" film stars of Bollywood to advise the public that soft drinks are safe. Isn't interesting?

Now let me summarise all the learning:

Habit No 1: If you are seriously interested in losing extra weight and gaining health then please, ensure that from this moment onwards **you are not going to drink soft drinks anymore**, for your own good health and switch to plain still water instead.

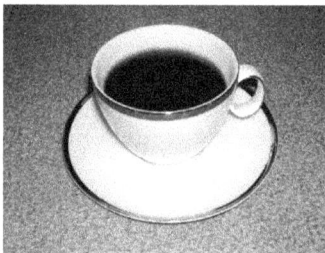

A Cappuccino, with whole milk 190 g drink can have 65 Kcal with 4 g fat.

A single cup of fresh coffee can give about 80-330 mg of caffeine per cup depending upon type of beans, the way coffee is made and how strong the brew is.

Food Habit No 2

Coffee

Drinking coffee is a social activity and is enjoyable as per current trend in our society. It certainly seems to provide a welcome break from work and other activities.

Now before I write the verdict on coffee let's first learn more about the main constituent in coffee which is known as caffeine.

Caffeine

Caffeine is a mild stimulant and one of the main constituent of coffee. Caffeine is mostly found in coffee, tea, soft drinks and chocolate.

Caffeine can make you feel more alert and awake. It can increase your heart rate and pulse. You can feel awake and alert - especially in the morning. If you take higher doses, it may prevent you from sleeping.

It is addictive and people tend to rely on it to give them a boost. It can also lead to withdrawal symptoms when stopped taking its consumption.

For example, if you decide to stop taking coffee there is very high possibility that you would experience headaches and drowsiness for couple of days.

Now let's see the statistics of drinking coffee in UK. You can see every day in the morning before office hours, coffee houses in London are certainly full. *In Britain about 70% of adults drink coffee and on average each person drinks 3.5 cups of coffee per day*[14] which is very high from my point of view.

What I am going to say now about coffee will definitely surprise you after all those great benefits you might have heard which are propagated by media about coffee.

If you drink too much coffee, it is certainly not good for your health.

Well, coffee contains caffeine and as you have read above the caffeine is addictive and it is one of the world's most widely used drugs which can be the cause of numbers of health problems. For example:

- It can prevent your body from absorbing vitamins and minerals.

- It can increase the excretion of vitamins and minerals from the body, so you may not get the full benefits of healthy foods.

- It can increase your heart rate and blood pressure.

- It has an impact on the body's energy levels: following the initial energy surge, the levels fall due to the lowering of blood sugar.
- It can cause headaches and insomnia and this is not all.

Coffee & Bad Breath

Have you ever smelt the breath of someone who is a heavy coffee drinker? It does not certainly smell nice.

Caffeine & Sleep

If you are having difficulties in sleeping check yourself if you are taking coffee before sleeping.

You would be surprised to know that caffeine could be one of the many reasons for disturbed sleep and of course disturbed sleep is certainly very unhealthy for overall health.

However, the effect of caffeine on sleep varies from person to person.

Caffeine and PMS

According to Jean Carper
Food: Your Miracle Medicine: How Food Can Prevent and Cure over 100 Symptoms and Problems:

"Those consuming at least one cup of a caffeine-containing beverage per day, such as coffee, tea or soft drinks, were more prone to PMS. And the more caffeine they consumed, the more severe their PMS symptoms." [9]

Habit No 2:

The second habit you need to develop now onwards is to **minimise your intake of caffeine** and best if you can altogether eliminate it from your food intake. Take plain still water instead.

If you cannot cut down on the number of cups of coffee then, cut down on the size of cups so you drink half the quantity.

Please make sure no more than one cup of coffee per day.

"When health is absent, wisdom cannot reveal itself, art cannot become manifest, strength cannot be exerted, wealth is useless and reason is powerless."

- Herophilies, 300 B.C.

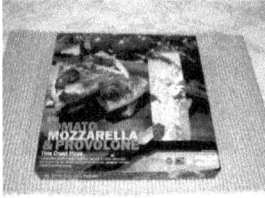

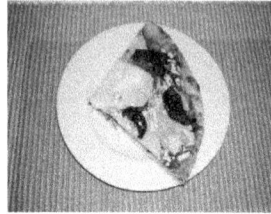

A Tomato Mozzarella & Provolone Pizza (V) of 330 g can have **730 Kcalories**, about **25 g fat** (11.6 g saturated) and 3.6 g of salt (**60 % of salt GDA**)

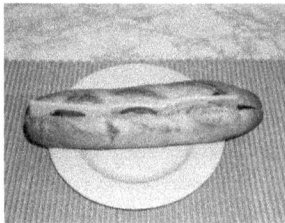

A Ploughman's baguette can provide **603 Kcal**, **23.5 g fat** (11.6 g saturated fat) and **3.7 g salt**

Food Habit No 3

Fast food

Next habit which is killing western nations is fast food.

As per news published on US department of health and human service, NIH news website " *Eating at Fast-food Restaurants More than Twice Per Week is Associated with More Weight Gain and Insulin Resistance in Otherwise Healthy Young Adults*" [15]

This extra weight puts you at risk for developing many diseases, especially heart disease, stroke, diabetes, and cancer, etc. So in a way fast food is helping you to gain weight and put you in danger of losing health.

According to other news on BBC News 24 titled "Why fast food makes you get fat" says that *"The nutritional make up of fast food encourages people to gorge on it unintentionally, increasing their risk of obesity, research suggests".*

It further explains that *"most fast food is very dense in calories - you only need a small amount to bump up your calorific intake.*

They found that these "energy dense" foods can fool people into consuming more calories than the body needs". "The *researchers concluded that a diet high in fast foods will increase a person's risk of weight gain and obesity - even though they may feel that they are eating no more than they would if they ate an average meal"*[16].

Consumption of Fast-food is certainly increasing in western nations over the past decades. If you look at nutritional value in the food at the fast food joints, you would be surprised to know that most of the food does not have any nutritional value despite some of their recent healthful offerings, the menus still tend to include foods high in fat, sugar and calories and low in fiber and nutrients. For example, a Tomato Mozzarella & Provolone Pizza (V) of 330 g can have **730 Kcalories**, about **25 g fats** which is very high and almost half of it saturated.

Now the question is: why do we eat all these fast food when it is not so healthy? Well, the reason perhaps may be that it tastes really good. Certainly it seems difficult to resist the temptation of burgers, pizza, French fries, etc but unfortunately indulging in fast food brings extra weight along with it. By the end of the day the choice is always ours.

Habit No 3:

If you are looking forward to lose weight, you need to develop habit no 3 which is **Avoid Fast Food**.

If you can't, then make sure you are watchful of what quantity you eat. Keep fast food only as a treat to yourself once in a while.

"You put a baby in a crib with an apple and a rabbit. If it eat the rabbit and plays with the apple, I will buy you a new car."

- Harvey Diamond

Food Habit No 4

Meat

I cannot overemphasise the point that meat is certainly not good for human health. If you are eating meat regularly, there is very high possibility that you would gain weight apart from developing issues related to digestion. Let's have a look at some of the following research reports on meat and weight gain.

As per study published on *Magazine* Physician committee for responsible medicine under titled "*Meat-Eaters Gain Weight*" "*A new study confirms that meat-eating encourages weight gain. Researchers from the American Cancer Society studied 79,236 young and middle-aged men and women, measuring their diets in 1982 and again in 1992. Those who ate more than three servings of meat per week were much more likely to gain weight as the years went by, compared to those who tended to avoid meat*". [17]

"We stopped eating meat many years ago. During the course of a Sunday lunch, we happened to look out of the kitchen window at our young lambs playing happily in the fields. Glancing down at our plates, we suddenly realised we were eating the leg of an animal who had until recently been playing in a field herself. We looked at each other and said "Wait a minute, we love these sheep - they're such gentle creatures. So why are we eating them?" It was the last time we ever did."

- Paul and Linda Mccartney

According to another news on website of **Cancer Research UK titled** "Switching to vegetarianism keeps weight down"

Cancer Research UK scientists studied the eating habits of 22,000 meat eaters, fish eaters, vegetarians and vegans of all ages over five years and compared weight gains in all these categories. According to them *"Meat-eaters who switch to vegetarianism gain less weight over a five year period than people who make no changes to their dietary habits"*[18]

According to news published on Vegetarian & Vegan Foundation UK, titled "Government Urged to Face-Up to Real Cause of Obesity":

"New research by the *Vegetarian & Vegan Foundation (VVF)* shows that meat and dairy are at the core of the world's expanding obesity epidemic..." *"The American Cancer Society followed 75,000 people over a decade and found that one food was most associated with weight gain – meat".*[19]

There are number of studies which have come out on ill effect of meat on health. Without going much into details I would like to highlight few out of many points:

- I do not find any nutrient which is absolutely necessary for human health which is found only in meat but not in plant food.
- Most of animal foods are higher in fat content than most plant foods, particularly saturated fats.
- Meat is largely deficient in vitamins except for the b-complex.

"As custodians of the planet it is our responsibility to deal with all species with kindness, love and compassion. That these animals suffer through human cruelty is beyond understanding. Please help stop this madness."

- Richard Gere

The fat content in meat is very high. You could be surprised to know that fat content in Lamb (breast, untrimmed, roasted) of 90 g average portion is about 27 g fat which is too high. Similarly about 100gms of meatloaf contains 11g of fat but *for a healthy weight loss diet, I would recommend that one should go for food which has fat content less than 5 %.*

Meat is very high in protein but have no fiber (which should be part of healthy diet).

"For weight loss or to maintain the healthy weight, one needs fiber rich food with less than 5 % fat content while meat contains about 10 to 20% fat without any fiber. Weight Loss program and meat cannot go together".

If you are a meat eater, I know you may be thinking that for every research I have quoted here, you can also suggest me some study showing positive benefits of eating meat. So let's consider following point and see if it makes sense to you.

How many times did you go to see a doctor when you fell ill? Unless people find themselves really ill, they take some medicine of their own. Now what do you think in the case of animals?

Do you think every time an animal is ill and the person whose sole purpose is to earn the money by killing them would spend money on their health? Unless the animal is really ill and this illness could seriously affect other animals and his profit margins too, the chances are very less that the owner will spend money every time, if any of them is unhealthy.

"The labels are misleading the public. The labels should declare that the product has been contaminated with fecal material...Today, nationwide, line speeds are up to 140 to 160 carcasses per minute. It's not humanly possible for meat inspectors to do what they are required to do, which is to protect the consumer."

-- Delmer Jones, President of the US Meat Inspector Union

Now this means that there is every possible chance that the meat which you could be eating with your dinner could have some sort of disease. Think for a second that your dinner which you perceive as healthy may not be healthy after all and disease could enter into your body.

Still thinking…? Ok, let's look from another aspect; the animal was killed in healthy condition.

Do you think before making the nice tasty sausage or ham, the intestine of animals are located precisely and then get cleaned from faeces, disinfected or eliminated for every animal, throughout the day, everyday round the year so that you may not end up eating animal s**t along with the flesh.???

Think for a moment you could be eating animal dead body which could be ill and dirty??? Still not convinced! Ok then read the following comments by-- Delmer Jones, President of the US Meat Inspector Union. *"The labels are misleading the public. The labels should declare that the product has been contaminated with fecal material…Today, nationwide, line speeds are up to 140 to 160 carcasses per minute. It's not humanly possible for meat inspectors to do what they are required to do, which is to protect the consumer."*

There is one more point I would like you to think from another dimension.

Our body is made up of the food we eat. Every food we eat brings some kind of qualities associated with the food in our body and also effect the state of our mind.

"The beef industry has contributed to more American deaths than all the wars of this century, all natural disasters, and all automobile accidents combined. If beef is your idea of 'real food for real people,' you'd better live real close to a real good hospital."

--Neal D. Barnard, M.D., President Physicians Committee for Responsible Medicine

For example, if you eat chillies you can instantly feel heat in your mouth and your mind will become agitated and if you practice meditation regularly you can even experience the impact of all kind of foods on your mind.

When you kill an animal, obviously the animal cannot be happy but sad and fearful. So when the animal is dying because of extreme sadness and fear, certain hormones are released into his body which also enter into your body when you eat them.

So now imagine whenever you eat the animal food you also eat the hormones of sadness and fear which at some level create various kind of diseases in human body.

I would like to explain, that the lack of awareness is natural if you were born in the family which include meat in their daily diet. So you were eating what your parents thought is healthy for you and you were brought up thinking that having a beef burger or ham sandwich is a natural way of living.

Now as an adult you have the choice to decide what is healthy for you.

Your right decision would certainly help you to lose weight and have healthy life forever.

Habit No 4:

You have to stop eating meat for your own good health.

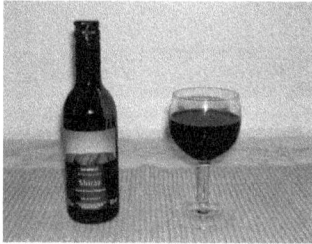

If you drink wine regularly even under the safe limit, still you may end up putting on at least 26 pounds of extra weight each year.

Food Habit No 5

Alcohol

Many times I came across people who ask me "Mr Gupta, I have been exercising regularly and eating healthily but still I can't shed those extra pounds". My answer always starts with asking them a question: how much alcohol they drink?

Perhaps it's time for you to look how much alcohol you drink. Considering the number of calories each drink has let's see how many calories you consume every week.

For example, if you are habitual of drinking 1 pint of beer a day (1 pint of beer about 182kcal) you would end up putting on extra 5460 k calories each month. Now 3500 calories approximately equal to one pound, which means you could be putting on approximately 1.5 pounds of extra weight each month and this would result in 18 pounds of extra body weight per year just by drinking 1 pint of beer a day.

Let's take another example; you drink about 3 units of red wine a day (*Safe limit for men as per advise of department of health UK*).

Now 3 units of red wine a day means about 255 empty k calories a day in your body (1 small glass 125ml of red wine has about 85 Kcal), which means 7650 k calories each month. That means you can easily put on 2.18 pounds each month which may result in 26.23 pounds of extra body weight each year just by drinking red wine under safe limit as per the guideline by UK govt.

Yes you have read it correctly "If you drink wine regularly even under the safe limit, still you may end up putting on at least 26 pounds of extra weight each year."

Now think what about those people who often drink beyond safe limits. Now imagine if you cut back on your alcohol drinks how much weight you could lose naturally.

Apart from losing weight, sensible drinking habits would also help to keep you away from liver disease.

Alcohol is a liquid and we can consume many more calories by sipping it for hours, without ever feeling full.

We often mix it with juice or soda which adds even more calories. But perhaps the worst effect alcohol has on our weight is that it removes our inhibitions, so we eat and drink much more than we need or plan to.

Few facts you would like to know about Alcohol:

- Alcohol helps fat to be absorbed effectively.

- Alcohol, especially white wine and champagne enhances your appetite. So if you drink it before the meal, surely you would end up eating more and hence the extra weight.

- Alcohol tends to dehydrate you and dehydration can slow your metabolism preventing weight loss.

Another point to consider is that Alcohol does not affect everyone the same way. Women and older people will generally be at greater risk of these effects even at lower levels of consumption.

Number of studies has been done on alcohol. Some of the studies show the health benefits of alcohol consumption *but only when you take it in moderation*. However, the issue is that alcohol is very addictive and most of the time people end up in excess drinking.

Excess drinking of alcohol has also been linked with some type of cancers, malnutrition because of changes in digestion and metabolism, muscle cramp, depression and osteoporosis, etc.

How many units?

The alcohol content of drinks is measured in units. One UK unit contains eight grams of pure alcohol.

UK Government department of health advises: Men should not regularly drink more than three to four units a day: 3-4/day; (@8g = 24-32g day) and women not more than two to three: 2-3/day; (@8g = 16-24g/day). Of course, in some situations like pregnancy, avoid drinking alcohol.

A pint 568ml of beer at 4% ABV contains 2.3 units,
White Wine at 12 % ABV (Medium - 175 ml):2.1 units,
Red wine at 8 % ABV (large, 250ml): 2.0 units,
25ml measure of vodka at 37.5 %: 0.9 Unit

Habit No 5

My recommendation for alcohol intake is different than the Heath Department advice. Habit no 5 is to make sure **never drink more than once a week and do not exceed 4 units.**

I know you might be thinking now: *"If I drink only 4 units I am not going to enjoy it."* I can assure you that you will have the same enjoyment within 4 units which you experience normally after 8 to 10 units because your body would be detoxified by following 7 habits described in this book.

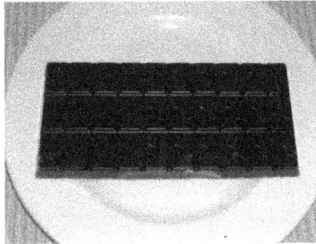

A smooth milk chocolate of 200g can provide **1082 Kcal**, **112 g sugar** and **64 g Fat (38 g Saturated Fat)**

Food Habit No 6

Chocolate/ Crisps

To anybody and everybody who is interested in losing weight, one thing needs to be clear that you need to get rid of products like chocolate and crisps. The chocolate has lots of calories is small portion because it is a dense calorie food. In fact chocolate / crisps not only contain many calories but also unhealthy fat and lots of sugar.

A potato crisp is a thin slice of potato, deep fried or baked. Some of us may think that crisps are healthy potatoes cooked in sunflower oil and is a perfect snack.

The reality is most crisps consist of *trans fat* and **masses of chemicals** and they are not natural as you may think. Many crisps are just mashed potato mix and a cocktail of additives.

Deep-frying is a cooking method whereby food is submerged in hot oil or fat.

Habit No: 6

Well, I would say that just **avoid Chocolate / Crisps** and if you cannot avoid them then please eat them as once in a while but certainly not as a regular snack.

"Nothing will benefit human health and increase chances for survival of life on Earth as much as the evolution to a vegetarian diet".

Albert Einstein

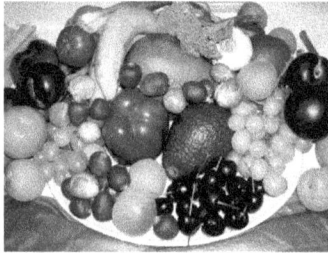

Apple 100g average portion can provide **43 kcal** and **only traces of fat.**

Banana 100 g average portion can provide **95 kcal** and **only 1 g fat.**

Orange 160 g average portion can provide **59 kcal** and **only traces of fat.**

Food Habit No 7

Fruits and vegetables

Are you interested in food which not only helps you to lose weight effectively but also helps in warding off heart disease and stroke, control blood pressure and cholesterol and prevent some types of cancer?

Welcome, you have reached healthy food Habit no 7: Fruits and Vegetables.

Make sure you eat lots of fruits and vegetables every day.

Fruits and vegetables would not only help you to lose weight but would also help you to avoid many diseases.

There are hundreds of research studies done which prove that fruits and vegetables are extremely good for the healthy life style.

According to information published on Harvard School of Public Health website titled "Fruits and Vegetable"

"Eating plenty of fruits and vegetables can help you ward off heart disease and stroke, control blood pressure and cholesterol, prevent some types of cancer, avoid a painful intestinal ailment called diverticulitis, and guard against cataract and macular degeneration, two common causes of vision loss." [20]

Similarly according to another article *"Scientific studies have shown that people who eat a lot of fruit and vegetables may have a lower risk of getting illnesses, such as heart disease and some cancers. For this reason, health authorities recommend that you eat at least five portions of fruit and vegetables every day."* [21]

Fruits and vegetables have many positive effects on our health:

• Their high fibre content helps control blood glucose levels, reduces cholesterol and probably reduces the risk of colon cancer and other cancers.

• They contain antioxidants which may reduce the risk of coronary heart disease.

• They contain essential vitamins and minerals that are vital for good health and disease prevention.

One of the beneficial components of fruits and vegetables is their fiber content. Fiber can calm the irritable bowel and relieve constipation.

How much do I need?

The general common advice in terms of eating fruits and vegetables is of five portions a day. However these five portions should come from a variety of sources every day. I would recommend at least eat 5 portions a day and *if you are interested in losing weight fast make it 8 to 10 portions a day.*

Fruits

To gain the maximum benefit from fruits, it is best to eat them fresh. I would recommend that it is better to eat fruits than drinking fruit juices because fruit loses most of its natural fibre in the juicing process.

One can eat at least two or three portions of fruit every day. One portion equal to 80gms:

• Apple, banana, pear or orange.

• 1/2 avocado

• 1 large slice of melon or fresh pineapple

• 3 dried apricots

• 1 cupful of grapes, cherries or berries

Vegetables

One can aim for at least two to three portions of vegetables each day. One portion equal to 80gms, which would be a

- 1 cereal bowl of lettuce

- 1 cereal bowl of salad

- 3 tablespoons of cooked carrots or peas or sweet corn, etc.

Eating plenty of fruits and vegetables is good for eyes. Vitamin A in carrots helps night vision. Fruits and vegetables also help in preventing two common aging-related eye diseases - cataract and macular degeneration - which afflict millions of people worldwide.

Fruits and vegetables are clearly an important part of a good diet. Everyone can benefit from eating them; however important point is variety along with quantity.

Habit No: 7

Everyday intake of fruits and vegetables should be at least 5 portions a day and if interested in weight loss, take 7 to 8 portions every day.

Follow these 7 habits for 6 weeks and please write to me your success story at: info@subodhgupta.com

Now after reading this whole book you must be wondering that millions of people worldwide eat all these products and all of them cannot be wrong so are all these people ignorant???

Well, the answer is the marketing of unhealthy products is so powerful that majority of people choose to buy those foods and most of the time we just assume that majority cannot be wrong; I eat and drink what everybody else does and everybody cannot be wrong.

For a moment let's consider this kind of approach is Ok but then why obesity is increasing like never before? Why so many people are falling ill and dying because of present day lifestyle diseases? Why is the health of advanced western nations failing (more than 100 million American have high cholesterol)?

Now you might be thinking, well there can be many other factors as well responsible for all these diseases. Yes you are right. There are combinations of factors which are responsible for ill health but point to emphasise here is our food is the most important aspect in all these factors.

If we take out unhealthy food habits and replace them with healthy one we will lose weight naturally and gain health forever without much effort.

The only way to live a healthy life and have perfect body weight is to have healthy eating and drinking habits.

Healthy Food Habits = Good Health + Perfect Body Weight *Forever*

Part 2

Recording Improvement

Wellness Monitor

Before beginning Food Habit plan, please take couple of minutes to fill in the following Wellness monitor.

	Wellness Monitor	
S.N.	Indicators	Before Beginning
1	Blood Pressure (High)	
	(Low)	
2	Hours of sleep (average per week)	
3	Quality of sleep (1 to 5) (1 lowest and 5 the best, average for the week)	
4	Body Weight	
5	Overall energy level (1 to 5) (1 lowest and 5 highest)	

Daily Food Habit Record

Week 1

Starting Date ……………………….

S.N.	Food Habits	Sun	Mon	Tue	Wed	Thu	Fri	Sat
1	Soft Drinks							
2	Coffee							
3	Fast Food							
4	Meat							
5	Alcohol							
6	Chocolate & Crisps							
7	Fruits & Vegetables							

Daily Food Habit Record

Week 2

S.N.	Food Habits	Sun	Mon	Tue	Wed	Thu	Fri	Sat
1	Soft Drinks							
2	Coffee							
3	Fast Food							
4	Meat							
5	Alcohol							
6	Chocolate & Crisps							
7	Fruits & Vegetables							

Daily Food Habit Record

Week 3

S.N.	Food Habits	Sun	Mon	Tue	Wed	Thu	Fri	Sat
1	Soft Drinks							
2	Coffee							
3	Fast Food							
4	Meat							
5	Alcohol							
6	Chocolate &Crisps							
7	Fruits & Vegetables							

Daily Food Habit Record

Week 4

S.N.	Food Habits	Sun	Mon	Tue	Wed	Thu	Fri	Sat
1	Soft Drinks							
2	Coffee							
3	Fast Food							
4	Meat							
5	Alcohol							
6	Chocolate& Crisps							
7	Fruits & Vegetables							

Daily Food Habit Record

Week 5

S.N.	Food Habits	Sun	Mon	Tue	Wed	Thu	Fri	Sat
1	Soft Drinks							
2	Coffee							
3	Fast Food							
4	Meat							
5	Alcohol							
6	Chocolate& Crisps							
7	Fruits & Vegetables							

Daily Food Habit Record

Week 6

S.N.	Food Habits	Sun	Mon	Tue	Wed	Thu	Fri	Sat
1	Soft Drinks							
2	Coffee							
3	Fast Food							
4	Meat							
5	Alcohol							
6	Chocolate & Crisps							
7	Fruits & Vegetables							

Wellness Monitor

After completing your 6 week healthy food habit plan, please take couple of minutes to fill in the following wellness monitor and compare that how you have improved on following parameters.

	Wellness Monitor	
S.N.	Indicators	After 6 week of
1	Blood Pressure (High)	
	(Low)	
2	Hours of sleep (average per week)	
3	Quality of sleep (1 to 5) (1 lowest and 5 the best, average for the week)	
4	Body Weight	
5	Overall energy level (1 to 5) (1 lowest and 5 highest)	

Reference:

(1)Department of Health, “Policy and Guidance: Obesity General Information”<online>
http://www.dh.gov.uk/en/Policyandguidance/Healthandsocialcaretopics/Obesity/DH_078098

(2)Foresight, “Our Work: Scoping the Foresight Project on Tackling Obesities, Future Choices”<online>
http://www.foresight.gov.uk/obesity/outputs/Scoping/Results_of_Scoping.html

(3) MSN UK "Life & style: Scotland is the second fattest nation"<online>
http://style.uk.msn.com/wellbeing/healthyeating/article.aspx?cp-documentid=6237321

(4)American Cancer Society, “Cancer Statistics 2007 Presentation ”<online>
http://www.cancer.org/docroot/PRO/content/PRO_1_1_Cancer_Statistics_2007_Presentation.asp

(5)Cancer Research UK, “News and Resources: UK cancer mortality statistics for common cancers”<online>
http://info.cancerresearchuk.org/cancerstats/mortality/cancerdeaths/

(6) Center for Science in public interest (CSPI), “Liquid Candy: How soft drinks are harming America’s health”<online>
http://www.cspinet.org/liquidcandy/

(7) Greenhalgh, Alyson, "Carbonated soft drinks" <online>
http://www.bbc.co.uk/health/healthy_living/nutrition/drinks_soft2.shtml

(8)United States National Institute of Diabetes and Digestive and Kidney Diseases (NIDDK), “Study Links Soft Drink Consumption to Childhood Obesity”<online>
http://win.niddk.nih.gov/notes/winnotesfall01/studylinkssoft.htm

(9)New Target, "The health effects of drinking soda - quotes from the experts" January 08, 2005 <online> http://www.newstarget.com/004416.html

(10)Harvard School of Public Health (HSPH), "Active Girls Who Drink Colas are Five Times More Likely to Fracture Bones "16th June 2000 <online> http://www.hsph.harvard.edu/ats/Jun16/june16_02.html

(11)Hickman, Martin, Independent News "Caution: Some soft drinks may seriously harm your health"27th May 2007 <online> http://news.independent.co.uk/health/article2586652.ece

(12)BBC News 24 "Health: Cancer chemical found in drinks" 1st March 2006 <online> http://news.bbc.co.uk/1/hi/health/4763528.stm

(13) Centre for Science and Environment (CSE), "Soft Drinks Still Unsafe" Press Release August 02, 2006 <online> http://www.cseindia.org/misc/cola-indepth/cola2006/cola_press2006.htm

(14) Leeds Student Medical Practice" Health Advice: Caffeine" <online> http://www.leeds.ac.uk/lsmp/healthadvice/caffeine/caffeine.htm

(15) US department of health and human service, National Institute of health "Eating at Fast-food Restaurants More than Twice Per Week is Associated with More Weight Gain and Insulin Resistance in Otherwise Healthy Young Adults" 30th December 2004 <online> http://www.nih.gov/news/pr/dec2004/nhlbi-30.htm

(16) BBC News 24 "Health: Why fast food makes you get fat" <online> http://news.bbc.co.uk/1/hi/health/3210750.stm

(17) The Physicians Committee for Responsible Medicine "Magazine, Obesity: Meat Eaters Gain Weight "autumn 1997 volume 6 number 4, <online>

http://www.pcrm.org/magazine/GM97Autumn/GM97Autumn12.html

(18) Cancer Research UK, Press Release Archive "Switching to vegetarianism keeps weight down" 14th March 2006 <online> http://info.cancerresearchuk.org/news/archive/pressreleases/2006/march/115425

(19) Vegetarian & Vegan Foundation "Write to Fight Flab: Government Urged to Face-Up to Real Cause of Obesity" <online> http://www.vegetarian.org.uk/campaigns/globesity/letters.html

(20) Harvard School of Public Health "Fruit and Vegetables" <online> http://www.hsph.harvard.edu/nutritionsource/fruits.html

(21) Stinton M, BBC Health "Fruits and Vegetables"<online> http://www.bbc.co.uk/health/healthy_living/nutrition/basics_fruitveg1.shtml

Our Published Books

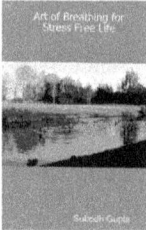

Art of Breathing *for* Stress free Life
The Only book on human breathing techniques for managing stress with clearly illustrated photographs and practical instructions. This book is ideal for busy people who lead a hectic life style.

ISBN 978-1-84799-047-1
Library of Congress Control Number: 2007907962
Soft cover /£9.95/ 56 pages

Gentle Yoga for 50 Plus

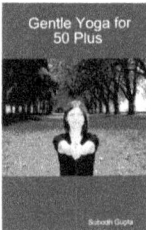

"A perfect gift of health for your parents"

The only book on Gentle Yoga for people in the age group of 50 plus. The exercises explained in this book are also beneficial if suffering from arthritis or rheumatism.

ISBN 978-1-84799-149-2,
Library of Congress Control Number: 2007908785
Soft cover/ £9.95/ 56 pages

For more details please visit our website:
www.subodhgupta.com/books.html

All our books are available on Amazon, Barnes and Nobles.

Simplified Yoga for Backache

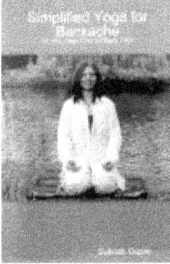

This book is a carefully designed practical guide for preventing and managing back pain.

Majority of back pain are caused by muscular insufficiency and lack of flexibility. A strong and flexible back creates the foundation for a healthy lifestyle.

Simplified yoga poses described in this book can be practiced by everybody, whether young or old, beginner or advanced. These poses will strengthen the back muscles and improve flexibility.

Page 68/ Soft cover/ £6.95
ISBN: 978-0-9556882-4-9

India Culture and Travel scams

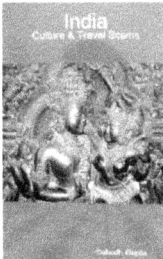

This is a practical book about understanding Indian culture and travel scams in India and is based on real life experiences.

This book will help you to avoid embarrassing mistakes and prepare you to feel confident in unfamiliar situations.

Content in this book includes Indian social customs, their perception about Western women, their religion, what motivates them, travel scams targeted at Western tourists and of course what not to discuss with Indians, etc.

Page 112/Paper Back / £7.95
ISBN 978-0-9556882-6-3

www.ingramcontent.com/pod-product-compliance
Lightning Source LLC
Chambersburg PA
CBHW022131280326
41933CB00007B/636